SAFE AND

PROVEN

DIABETES CURE

Scientifically proven Diabetes cure A~Z in 3 weeks, Insulin Resistance, Controlling Blood Sugar Levels, Weight Loss, Diabetes Meal Plan, Diabetes Exercise Plan

Christopher J. Davis, M.D.

Anna G Taylor

Table of Contents

INTRODUCTION

Congratulations on downloading *Safe and Proven Diabetes* Cure and thank you for doing so.

The following chapters will discuss everything about diabetes: whether you have just recently been diagnosed or are at risk for the disease, these pages will give you a full rundown of common myths, prevention methods, symptoms, and more. By the end of the book, you will have a fuller understanding of diabetes and the best way to treat it.

There are plenty of myths circulating that suggest that diabetes is always a consequence of poor eating habits and little physical activity, but this is not always the case. There are also a number of genetics and other uncontrollable environmental factors that many people do not know about, but here, we'll learn about what these can be and how you can prevent yourself from getting diabetes if you feel you are at risk.

Once you have learned about the disease, you will learn about how meditation and exercise can help you or your loved one keep diabetes in check. With a full guide on creating a workout, you'll know exactly how to design an exercise plan that works for you. Or, you can read about the benefits of yoga and meditation for diabetes (and stress!).

The final chapter of the book is dedicated to great vegan recipes for diabetics, with a full explanation of the benefits of veganism for diabetes. You'll be able to impress your friends with your simultaneously delicious and healthy cooking skills, and start to reverse the effects of diabetes on the body.

There are plenty of books on this subject on the market, so thanks again for choosing this one! Every effort was made to ensure that it is full of as much useful information as possible. Please enjoy!

Chapter 1: Myths About Diabetes

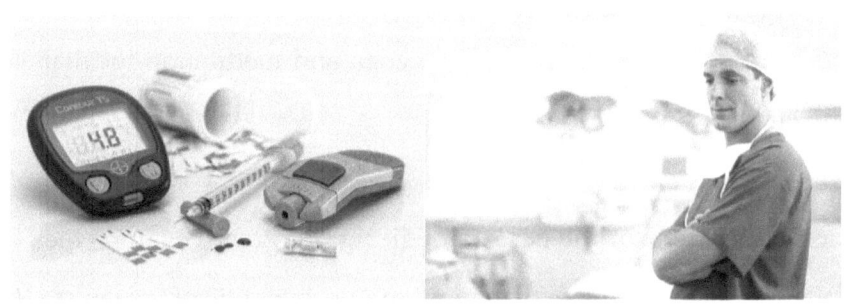

Being diagnosed with diabetes is difficult enough for patients without trying to sift through a bunch of myths perpetuated by pop culture and society at large. Whether you have, gestational diabetes, prediabetes, gestational diabetes, Type 1 or Type 2, there happens to be a wealth of information about diabetes to be found online and elsewhere. In the wake of a diagnosis, however, it can be overwhelming to sort out the good information from the bad.

Indeed, without some form of guidance, understanding what to expect with a diabetes diagnosis can be quite difficult. It doesn't help that pop culture is littered with myths about diabetes, some of which are based in truth and some of which have no facts behind them at all. For anyone who is recently suffering through a diagnosis of diabetes, or even prediabetes, trying to find the real information can be completely terrifying.

Unfortunately, it can also be a shame-inducing experience, because many people still believe that the sole factor in getting diabetes is obesity and physical activity. This is simply not true, and no one should be blamed for getting diabetes. In this first chapter, we will look at some of the myths about diabetes and debunking the ones that are just not true.

Causes of Diabetes

Despite a wealth of research on diabetes, there is very little conclusive evidence of diabetes being caused by any one particular thing. Unfortunately, however, there is no shortage of myths about the causes of diabetes. The problem with these sorts of myths is that is unnecessarily instills fear in people of the disease without any real basis in fact, and does not properly inform those who may actually be at risk for diabetes.

SAFE AND PROVEN DIABETES CURE

For example, one of the most common myths circulating about diabetes is that it is caused by increased sugar intake or obesity. While both of these things can be risk factors of diabetes, they are not by themselves the sole cause of diabetes. Since diabetes is a condition of the metabolic system provoked by the pancreas's failure to either produce or even use insulin effectively, obesity and increased sugar intake do have an effect on the progression of the disease. However, it is generally accepted that there is a genetic component to diabetes. People who get some form of diabetes are often thought to have a predisposition to it, which is then activated by some factor in the environment.

To be more specific, however, Type 2 diabetes is more often regarded as being genetic and linked to family history, while Type 1 diabetes requires that both parents carry certain risk factors for the disease. Some evidence to support that diabetes is genetic is the fact that Type 1 diabetes seems to be more prevalent in whites than other races. However, because this does not explain why people who are at risk do not always get the disease, research generally believes that some environmental factor triggers the onset of the disease.

The numbers of environmental factors that have been researched are many, but it could be anything from a virus to childhood diet, or some combination of many of these. Lifestyle certainly plays a role, and because families tend to have similar lifestyles, it is difficult to separate what is truly family history from what is simply a lifestyle choice.

Diet with Diabetes

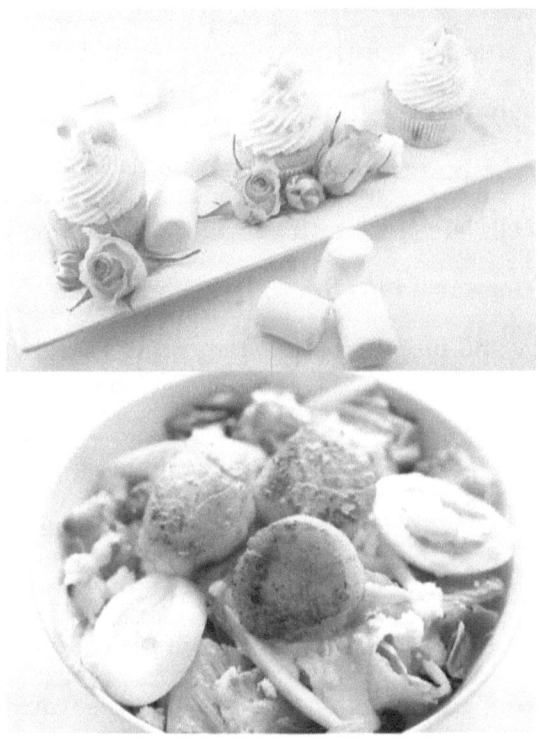

SAFE AND PROVEN DIABETES CURE

Another common myth about diabetes is that having it means that you will need to give up a wide variety of foods, most notably foods that tend to have a lot of sugar (like sweets and fruit). However, this is not always the case. Unsurprisingly, the key to a diet with diabetes is simply balance and moderation. You do not necessarily need to buy special diabetic foods or hold off on your favorite foods in order to live with the disease.

The biggest problem with eating as a diabetic is simply understanding and balancing the insulin in your body. Because you are unable to produce your own insulin with diabetes, your body cannot effectively use the food it eats. Even though you may eat a meal that would normally provide a lot of energy for a normal person, your cells are unable to use the glucose obtained from the meal because there is no insulin to transport it to the cells. You may still feel hungry and fatigued, even after eating a large meal.

What this means is that dieting on diabetes is a matter of glucose maintenance. You will likely have to monitor your blood-glucose levels before and after eating, and be aware of what happens if you have too much or too little insulin in your body. Hyperglycemia (elevated glucose) and hypoglycemia (low glucose) are the two major conditions that can occur without insulin maintenance, and both have their own set of symptoms that are serious in their own right.

So you do not necessarily need to completely abstain from eating cookies or your favorite fruits, but you do need to make sure that your body is able to use the energy that comes from the food you eat. Often, you can do this by working with a competent dietician to establish a meal plan that addresses your energy needs alongside your personal preferences.

Caring for Diabetes

One commonly known treatment for diabetes is insulin shots, which are used to artificially increase the level of insulin in the body to deal with the increased levels of blood-glucose. The myth about insulin shots is that having to take them is somehow a failure of the patient to properly maintain their diabetes. However, this is not necessarily the case.

Type 2 diabetes, for example, tends to be a progressive disease that gets worse over time, even if patients are trying to maintain it through oral medication, dieting, or exercise. The beta cells in the pancreas often simply stop producing insulin entirely as Type 2 diabetes progresses. For this reason, it is not a failure to have to take insulin shots. They should be thought of as a good thing that enables you to live your life more completely.

The biggest problem with myths about diabetes is that it makes it difficult for those who are seeking legitimate information about the disease to fully learn about it. Especially for recently-diagnosed diabetics, it can be very overwhelming to try to learn about the disease when a large portion of what you read is misleading and sometimes downright fake. In spite of these circulating myths, however, there are some legitimate strategies to preventing diabetes that you can implement in your daily life if you believe that you are at risk.

Preventing Diabetes

There are several factors associated with diabetes, including some associated with genetics. Despite this, there are plenty of steps you can take to prevent this condition from developing. Being diagnosed with prediabetes does not put an end to the world as you know it, even if you are at risk of developing the fully-fledged diseases– with some lifestyle changes, you can easily reverse the onset and continue to live a full and healthy life.

As we learned earlier, many people simply assume that the sole cause of diabetes is due to bad diet and exercise habits. Unfortunately, this puts a mantle of shame on the diagnosis of diabetes, and is not conducive to helping people get better. While obesity and inactivity can certainly be contributing factors to diabetes, there are also genetic and environmental factors (such as viruses).

For example, diabetes has a very strong genetic component. If one of your family members has diabetes, you are at a greater risk of having the disease. Make sure you know your family history so you know whether or not you should be careful with certain environmental factors, like your diet and exercise program. If diabetes is a disease that runs in your family, you might want to make sure that you eat healthy and exercise regularly preemptively.

SAFE AND PROVEN DIABETES CURE

Preventing diabetes is just a matter of setting concrete goals and making sure you meet them. You can't always control some of your risk factors, but you can definitely control setting goals to change your daily habits. Make sure that the goals you set for decreasing your blood-glucose level is realistic and has a clear pathway to achievement before setting it, otherwise it is easy to become discouraged and miss your goal.

When you set a goal, you should always make sure that it is specific enough that you know whether or not you have achieved it. For example, one great goal for preventing diabetes could be to order smaller portion sizes than you would normally. If, for example, you are going out to eat at a restaurant, maybe instead order a half-size of a meal. This is a specific goal. If you do not have realistic and specific goals, it can be harder to reach them.

Or, for example, another risk factor for diabetes is smoking. One goal to improve your lifestyle could be to quit smoking, which you could then break down into even smaller goals. By taking the larger task and making it into smaller ones, you will have a much easier time meeting your goal. Instead of just making a goal to quit smoking, you could start with not having a cigarette for a week. Or, alternatively, you could resolve to buy yourself the patch.

Aside from setting goals, you should also make a conscious effort to eat healthier and exercise. According to the Diabetes Prevention Program, for example, if someone with a high risk of diabetes lost even 5-7% of their total body weight, they could seriously decrease their risk of getting the disease. All this would require would be about 150 minutes of physical activity per week – something that can easily be broken into 30 minutes per day.

In later chapters, we will also be learning about healthy dieting and eating practices for diabetics, so even if you do not have diabetes, reading these chapters could help you figure out a plan to prevent the onset of diabetes if you are at risk.

Chapter 2: All About Diabetes: Symptoms, Types, and Solutions

Earlier in the book, we talked about common myths surrounding diabetes and the harmful effects that these myths can have on the diabetic populace. Then, we walked through some great prevention methods in order to help those who do not have the disease get their life back on track so that they are not at risk for having it. Here, we will be talking about how diabetes works biologically.

Without understanding properly what is happening in your body, it is difficult to make any sort of lifestyle change to improve diabetes. That's why we'll be walking through the ins and outs of diabetes on a purely biological level.

How Diabetes Works on a Biological Level

What is glucose?

Glucose is a simple sugar released by carbohydrate-rich foods like fruit, bread, and potatoes. Once consumed, these foods are broken down in the stomach, and the released glucose then travels to the intestines and then into your bloodstream. From your bloodstream, glucose then travels to the various cells in your body that need it for fuel (alongside amino acids and fats).

If your body has an excess of glucose, it is then stored in the liver and muscles in units called glycogens. Your body can store up to a day's worth of fuel in this way. When your blood-glucose levels become low, alpha cells in the liver produce a hormone called glucagon that breaks down glycogen into glucose to use for energy.

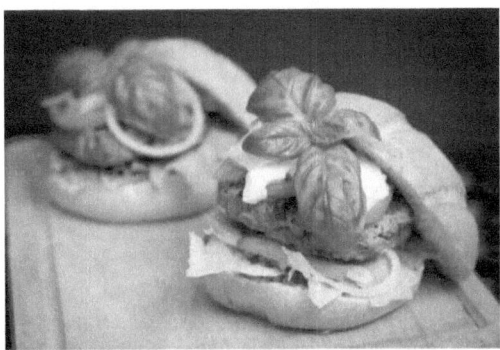

What is insulin?

Insulin is a hormone produced by beta cells in the pancreas. It allows the body to process the sugars (glucose) contained by the carbohydrates in the food you consume. Once insulin has itself attached to released glucose, it can then be used either directly for energy or stored for later. Insulin transports glucose to the cells that utilize it for fuel. Sugars that are not used immediately for energy are then stored in the liver for use at a later time when your body's blood glucose level is low (between meals, during physical activity, etc.). Insulin also prevents the liver from creating its own glucose in response to the level of glucose currently in your body.

Without insulin, your body cannot process glucose properly, and your blood sugar level increases because the sugars are not being converted into energy or stored as glycogens. This is called hyperglycemia.

What is hyperglycemia?

Hyperglycemia is a condition in which blood glucose levels are too high, causing a variety of symptoms, most notably increased urination, thirst, and hunger. It is the defining characteristic of diabetes and prediabetes. If hyperglycemia occurs outside of diabetes, it is usually treated based on the underlying cause of the condition.

Normal blood-glucose levels vary, but in general, above 70 milligrams per deciliter (mg/dL) up to around 125 mg/dL is considered normal, depending on whether or not you have recently eaten. This will, of course, vary from person to person. Blood-glucose levels will be increased directly following a meal. This is called reactive or postprandial hyperglycemia. You should consult your doctor to determine what normal blood-glucose levels are for you.

While hyperglycemia is generally regarded as a signature of diabetes, there are other conditions, which can cause it. Pancreatitis, pancreatic cancer, hyperthyroidism, and other medical conditions can also cause hyperglycemia. It can be a side effect of taking various medications or of elevated stress. Long-term hyperglycemia can cause a range of other medical problems and complications, many of which are evident in diabetes.

What is diabetes?

Diabetes (or diabetes mellitus) is a metabolic disease associated with high levels of blood sugar (specifically, glucose) causing frequent urination, thirst, hunger, weight gain or loss, fatigue, slow healing, numbing or tingling in the extremities, and sexual dysfunction. There are other symptoms of diabetes, all associated with the increased level of blood glucose. These high levels of blood sugar are caused by the body's inability to either produce or process insulin properly (or both).

An increased blood-glucose level eventually leads to long-term symptoms and complications.

Types of Diabetes

Though diabetes is a prominent health concern internationally, many people do not even know the difference between prediabetes, gestational diabetes, and the two types of diabetes (namely Type 1 and 2). Even though they are different, all of them have a similar effect on the body, each different type seems to be linked to a different cause.

Prediabetes

Prediabetes is a condition in which blood-glucose levels are abnormally high, but not yet high enough for a diagnosis of diabetes. Generally, prediabetes is heralded as a warning sign for Type 2 diabetes. Without changes in lifestyle, prediabetes can easily progress into Type 2. The cause the same as the cause of Type 2 diabetes – your body begins to develop insulin resistance or does not produce enough insulin.

As your body becomes unable to use insulin effectively or produce enough, you may begin to have symptoms of diabetes, such as hyperglycemia. Some people, however, have no symptoms of diabetes with prediabetes, which can make it more difficult to catch early on. Regardless of whether you have symptoms or not, a blood-glucose test in some form is necessary for an actual diagnosis of diabetes.

Type 1 Diabetes

Type 1 diabetes is the less common form of the disease, and was previously known as juvenile diabetes because it is normally diagnosed in children and young adults (though it can be diagnosed in persons over 20). According to the American Diabetes Association, only 5% of diagnosed cases of diabetes are Type 1 diabetes. Type 1 diabetes is characterized by the body's complete inability to produce insulin due to the destruction or damage of the beta cells in your pancreas.

Most commonly, this happens when your immune system targets islets of cells in the pancreas (3,000 to 4,000 cells) containing beta cells because it mistakenly views them as potential threats to your body. Beta cells are tasked with maintaining blood-glucose levels in the body and producing insulin when blood-glucose levels become high. When these cells are destroyed, the body becomes unable to produce insulin on its own. Without the insulin required to process glucose, it builds up in the bloodstream and cells are starved of the energy they need.

It is currently unknown why the immune system targets beta cells in type 1 diabetes. Generally, however, type 1 diabetes is treated with insulin shots. The problem with this, unfortunately, is balancing insulin intake with lifestyle. If too little insulin is taken, the long-term effects of hyperglycemia can cause complications. If too much insulin is taken, the body burns through the fuel and can cause hypoglycemia (low blood-glucose level). Hypoglycemia can be lethal if untreated.

Type 2 Diabetes

Type 2 diabetes is the far more common form of the disease, claiming at least 90% of cases. Unlike Type 1 diabetes, Type 2 is caused not by the body's inability to produce insulin at all, but rather by the body's resistance to insulin. Insulin resistance is simply when your body does not use the insulin produced by the pancreas properly. To make up for this resistance, the pancreas, then proceeds to produce even more insulin, but over time, cannot keep up with this production level.

With production of insulin being low or non-existent, the body is unable to utilize the energy from the foods you eat because the insulin is no longer there to transport the glucose into the cells that need it most.

SAFE AND PROVEN DIABETES CURE

Gestational Diabetes

Gestational diabetes is diabetes during pregnancy in women who have never had diabetes. Similar to Type 2 diabetes, gestational diabetes is initially caused by the body's resistance to insulin. It is thought that this is because the hormones produced by the placenta to facilitate the growth of a child can block insulin from being utilized properly. In response, the pancreas can produce up to three times more insulin than the mother would regularly need.

The American Diabetes Association states the prevalence of gestational diabetes as high as 9.2%. However, unlike Type 1 or Type 2 diabetes, gestational diabetes does not cause early birth defects because it emerges in late pregnancy. Despite this, a lack of proper maintenance can produce complications for both mother and child in gestational diabetes.

For example, when the mother's body cannot properly utilize insulin, the extra glucose in the bloodstream crosses the placenta to the baby. In response, the baby's pancreas will produce extra insulin to use up the glucose, but when it cannot, the glucose is stored as fat. This causes what is known as macrosomia, which can lead to a host of other problems for the child. Gestational diabetes can put the infant at an increased risk for breathing problems at birth and Type 2 diabetes later in life.

Symptoms of Prediabetes and Diabetes

As stated earlier, diabetes is caused by the way the body handles insulin, whether it is resistant to the hormone or unable to produce enough of it. No matter the type of diabetes, the symptoms are basically the same.

Increased Hunger and Fatigue

Without insulin, the body is unable to process the glucose contained in the food you eat. Because the glucose is used as fuel for your cells, when this glucose cannot enter them, they do not receive the energy they need. This causes a feeling of tiredness and hunger, often in spite of the fact that you have just eaten or are currently eating.

Increased Urination and Thirst

SAFE AND PROVEN DIABETES CURE

Most people will urinate anywhere from four to ten times a day, depending on a number of factors. Those with diabetes, however, will have to urinate more frequently due to the excess of glucose in their body. Though their function in glucose homeostasis is lesser known, the kidneys also perform a vital duty in balancing blood-glucose levels by reabsorbing glucose into the body. If there is too much glucose, the kidneys cannot keep up, and will instead try to get rid of the extra sugar by creating more urine.

Thus, those with diabetes will have an increased need to urinate and will often have more urine. Because urination requires fluids, it will in turn cause you to feel dehydrated and thirsty. This can then cause other issues, like dry skin or mouth.

Blurry Vision

Because diabetes so heavily affects the fluids in your body, one of the earliest noticeable symptoms of the disease is blurry vision. Blurry vision can be caused by fluids seeping into the eye, or by the thickness of blood with elevated levels of glucose present.

Slow Healing

Due to the increased viscosity of blood with high levels of glucose, it becomes more difficult for the body to circulate blood, which means that if you are wounded in any way (whether it be a minor cut, scrape, or bruise), your body has a more difficult time transporting blood to the affected area. Because of this, your body will heal itself much more slowly. Without proper treatment, these kinds of wounds can eventually lead to amputation.

Numbness and Tingling in the Extremities

One of the long-term symptoms of diabetes is increased numbness or tingling in the hands and feet. Similarly to slow healing, this is caused by the eventual nerve damage (neuropathy) to the body caused by long-term high levels of glucose in the bloodstream.

How Diabetes is Diagnosed

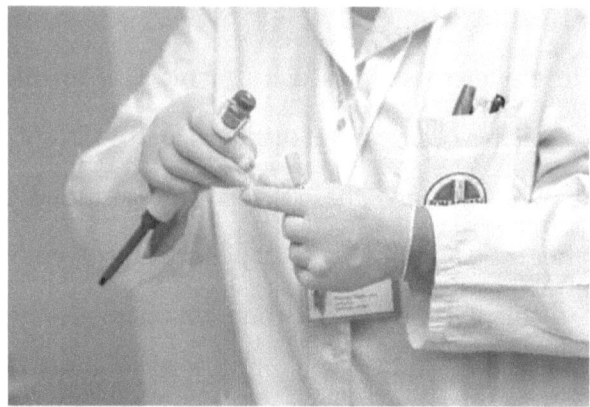

Diabetes is diagnosed through a variety of tests. Most of the time these tests need to be completed more than once for diabetes to be properly diagnosed, since the major determining factor of diabetes is the level of glucose in the body. Some of these tests must be taken before or after a meal so that there is some context for a blood-glucose level. If you have just eaten a meal, naturally there will be more glucose in your bloodstream as your body begins to transport the sugar to your cells for energy. If it has been a while since you last ate, your glucose level may be at a more balanced point as your body tries to remain in homeostasis.

Some of the tests for diabetes are as follows:

The A1C Test

The A1C blood test determines your average blood-glucose level over a period of two or three months by measuring the percentage of your red blood cells are coated with sugar. These cells are called glycated, and the higher the measurement of glycated cells, the higher the risk of diabetes. Normal A1C test results fall below 5.7%. Diabetes is diagnosed at a level of 6.5% or more.

This test is also used by doctors to monitor the blood-glucose levels of diabetics so that they are better able to maintain their glucose intake and insulin levels in the course of their treatment.

The Oral Glucose Tolerance Test (OGTT)

The Oral Glucose Tolerance Test is actually a series of blood tests over a short period of time that determines how your body handles glucose. In a span of 2 hours, your fasting glucose level will be measured as a baseline, and then your glucose level after consuming a sugary drink will be measured. The comparison between these two measurements and how the level changes over time are then studied.

Normal blood-glucose levels after 2 hours should fall below 140 mg/dL, and anything above 200 mg/dL is diagnosed as diabetes. In cases of gestational diabetes, this is the test most often used.

The Fasting Plasma Glucose Test

On the opposite end of the spectrum, the fasting plasma glucose test measures your blood-glucose levels following a fast. A fast in this context is defined as not having anything to eat or drink over a period of eight hours. For most patients, the test is performed first thing in the morning before any meals. After a fast, blood-glucose levels below 100 mg/dL are considered normal, while anything above 125 mg/dL is diagnosed as diabetes.

For any test, blood-glucose levels that fall between the normal and diabetes range is grounds for a diagnosis of prediabetes. Prediabetes can be treated before developing into Type 1 or 2 with changes in lifestyle.

Complications of Diabetes

A number of complications can arise from untreated or poorly managed diabetes, all of which, of course, stem from the body's increased blood-glucose levels.

Nerve Damage or Neuropathy

With the increased viscosity of your blood, it becomes more difficult for your body to transport it where it is needed. For this reason, patients with diabetes can eventually suffer nerve damage. Nerve damage is characterized by symptoms such as numbness or tingling in the extremities, most commonly in the feet.

The feet suffer a lot of damage as we walk around on them all day, and, often, wear poorly fitting shoes. Nerve damage to the feet is extremely serious because it completely disables them from self-maintaining, first because the nerves do not work, and second because they cannot feel when maintenance is needed.

Because you cannot feel your feet, many patients can hurt

themselves in some way and be unable to detect the pain or damage to the foot. Since blood is already not circulating to the area, wounds will be slower to heal. This can eventually lead to infection, which causes further damage to the foot, and if left untreated for a long period of time, can mean that amputation is required.

Nerve damage also means that your foot may be unable to monitor and control the condition of the skin surrounding it, so instead of producing the oil and moisture that it needs, the nerves stop working entirely. Calluses and ulcers can often build up because of the condition of the skin, which can also eventually lead to amputation.

Solutions for Diabetes

Regrettably, there is no such a thing as a hard and fast cure for this condition like there is antibiotics for infection. It can often be a lifetime disease, but with proper management, it can be effectively staved off so that patients are able to live out a full life. Some common solutions for diabetes are insulin injections, oral medications, and planned exercise and dieting. In the following chapters, we will discuss primarily meditation, exercise, and diet as a method for treating diabetes. Often, these solutions can greatly reduce the complications and symptoms of diabetes.

However, with the help of a good exercise plan, anyone can start to reverse the onset of diabetes. For example, three women treated by Dr. Christopher J. Davies managed to reverse their own diabetes by sticking to a healthy meal plan and exercise. By reminding themselves that their bodies needed the healthy food (instead of the junk they had previously been consuming), they were able to stay motivated in order to reverse the onset of the disease.

If you are trying to prevent or reverse the onset of diabetes, consider what makes you motivated. Do you have children? Do you have big dreams that you are afraid you won't be able to reach because of the disease? Try to make a list of the things that really motivate you, and every time you don't want to eat healthy or want to skip your exercise program, think of the things that motivate you. You can even write them down in a journal, or put them on sticky notes throughout your home.

SAFE AND PROVEN DIABETES CURE

All you really need to do in order to manage diabetes is be willing to make a serious lifestyle change, whether your diabetes is caused by genetic or environmental factors.

Chapter 3: Mindfulness and Diabetes

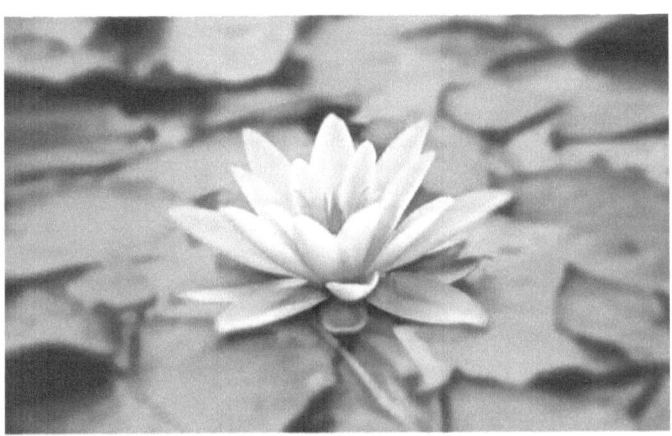

Among the many treatments for diabetes, one that is lesser known is mindfulness. You may have heard about using mindfulness for a variety of other mental and physical problems, but it can also be used to great effect to reduce the stress on the body for diabetes patients as well as uplift their mood. Even though it is a very serious disease, mindfulness can be very useful in helping both your mind and body get through the transition so that you can begin to live out your life more fully.

About Mindfulness

Historically, mindfulness has been practiced in Buddhism, where it is called sati (Pali) or smrti (Sanskrit). Sati is the first of Buddhism's "Seven Factors of Enlightenment", which is remembrance of the dharmas. However, the usage of mindfulness today is not quite the same as the usage of sati in Buddhism.

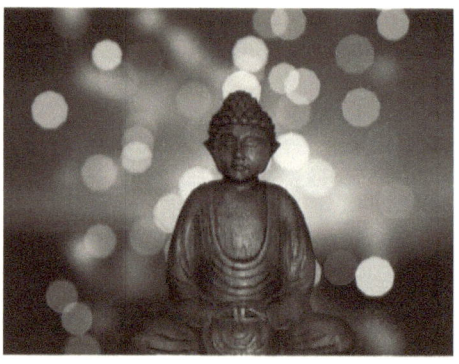

At its core, mindfulness is a state of mind that is achieved by being fully and completely in the present moment without being too reactive or overwhelmed. Today, it is primarily known as a psychological technique whereby patients redirect their attention away from their thoughts and instead focus on the world around them. However, this does not necessarily mean fully ignoring those thoughts, but instead coming to accept them. It is used often in psychology due to its proven effects in treating mental illnesses such as depression and anxiety.

Christopher J. Davis, **M.D.** /Anna G Taylor

Depression and anxiety are conditions that are often exacerbated by ruminating on unpleasant or negative thoughts – whether this be about oneself, the future, current circumstances, or more. Mindfulness in psychology is used to refocus a patient's attention to the world around them, enabling them to be more aware of their surroundings instead of merely focusing on the thoughts that cause depression and anxiety.

The most touted trait of mindfulness is simply "paying attention", and while this is indeed the core of the practice, there are other factors that must be considered during the practice of mindfulness. For example, another key component of mindfulness practice is non-judgment, which simply means being able to observe yourself and the world around you without judging it as either negative or positive. For most people, this is an incredibly difficult task. We are all predisposed and then subsequently trained into categorizing our experiences of the world as either "good" or "bad", and we have very little experience in non-judgment and letting go.

As such, mindfulness should not simply be thought of as a heightened level of awareness. It is a state of observation that prevents reactionary emotions and behaviors. Being very aware of a situation, but then judging it to be negative and reacting to it that way is not a practice of mindfulness. Letting go of experiences that we do not wish to have is a core element of mindfulness that is often overlooked, but no less important for it.

In combination with a heightened awareness of the world around us and ourselves in it, mindfulness then becomes more of a practice of "live and let live". It is adapting to the external world in a way that allows us to be more balanced internally. Mindfulness has become a bit of a buzz word today, but this is because its benefits are far-reaching. These include:

- Less rumination on depression and anxiety-inducing thoughts
- Lower overall stress levels
- Increased memory and focus
- Greater mood stability and less reactivity
- Development of self-observation and awareness

In today's world, who wouldn't want to become less stressed and have greater emotional satisfaction? Mindfulness is beneficial to just about everyone, including those with diagnosed with diabetes.

Practicing Mindfulness

Mindfulness is most often practiced in meditation, though it can be implemented as a passive skill with lots of practice. The first step to utilizing mindfulness in your daily life is paying attention to yourself and the world around you.

Find a place that is comfortable for you, whether it be in your own bedroom, in your car, or anywhere else. You may sit or stand. If you sit, it is better to sit cross-legged with your back straight and forming a right angle with the floor. Once you have settled in, take a deep breath, and begin to notice the world around you. Slowly allow your worries to fade away as you focus on your breathing.

Once you have reached a state of calm, observe your world and thoughts. Try to look at things without judgment, either good or bad. Observe your reactions to external stimuli. Do you become anxious or depressed very easily in reaction to your environment? Rather than feeling overwhelmed, try to instead take in the world around you without feeling good or bad.

One great way to observe your feelings is to visualize where in your body that feeling is coming from, and then note what that feeling is and save them for later. You do not need to act on it now, merely observe that it is there and that it will still be there if you want to act on it later. Continue observing the world around you. What do you notice about it?

You can easily catalog your observations in a journal when you are first getting started with mindfulness so you can learn what it is to be fully in your present moment. If you find your mind wandering, gently nudge it back to the present and continue the exercise. Mindfulness is all about being fully aware of and present in the current moment – it takes quite a bit of practice, so do not feel bad if you can't seem to slow your racing mind for very long.

You can practice mindfulness in a variety of different settings as well – in fact, you do not even need to fully meditate mindfully to practice the tenants of mindfulness. It can be hard to set aside time to meditate, especially if you are busy with work, kids, dieting, and more. In everyday life, however, you can still utilize mindfulness even if you do not have time for full meditation sessions.

No matter where you are, always make a conscious effort to be mindful. What are your surroundings like? What stands out to you? How do you feel about the world around you? By becoming more aware of yourself and your place in the world, you can reduce your stress levels, which ultimately exacerbate diabetes. As we saw earlier, mindfulness also has a host of other great benefits – whether you decide to implement it as a treatment for diabetes or for something else, mindfulness is a technique that everyone should learn.

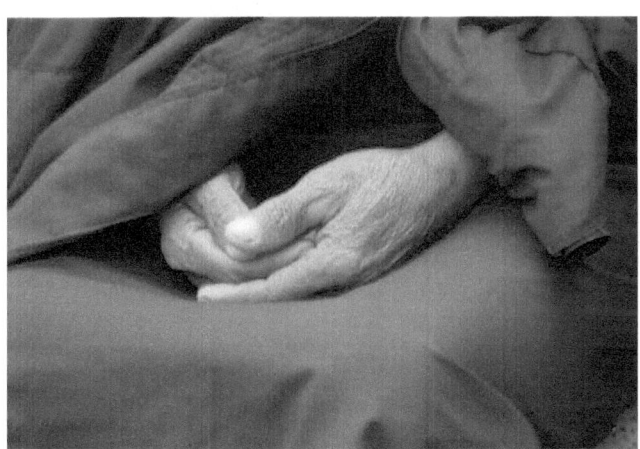

Chapter 4: Exercise for Diabetes

Exercise is a common suggestion for diseases and illnesses all across the board, including diabetes. If you go to a doctor and tell them that you are having trouble sleeping, one of the likely solutions that you will receive is to exercise more regularly. For some of us, exercise is a difficult time commitment, and it can be tough to get in shape. But the benefits of exercise on health are apparent, and certainly worth working for.

General Health Benefits of Exercise

There are plenty of benefits of regular exercise on health. Most people think of it as a way to lose weight, but that's not necessarily the only thing that it is used for. Exercise is also an effective way to combat mental illness such as depression and anxiety. The hormones released during physical activity are a great boost to happiness, and act as a natural antidepressant. That's why people who have depression are so often counseled to try to incorporate exercise into their routine.

Aside from the mental health benefits, however, there are some clear benefits for your body as well. Of course, the obvious ones are that you will lose weight and become more fit and physically in shape, but there are other not so obvious ones. For one, if you do not already have diabetes, exercise is one way to lessen your chance for it.

However, exercise also reduces the risk of suffering from other life-threatening and life-long diseases, included but not limited to heart disease. It is estimated that around 1 in 4 people each year will die from heart disease in the United States. This particular condition is actually the primary cause of death in the whole world, more so than cancer. With just a little exercise, however, your risk of heart disease goes down significantly.

Exercise also strengthens the body's natural circadian rhythm, which means that if you exercise regularly for long enough, you will get more and better quality sleep. It also helps increase energy levels. This may seem counterintuitive, since you have to expend energy to exercise, but in fact, lower intensity exercise programs can give you a boost of energy and lower how fatigued you feel.

People who exercise often have also been shown to have a better memory and performance at their everyday tasks, like work and school. Overall, exercise is a great way to live a healthier and more full life.

How to Create an Exercise Plan to Combat Diabetes

Even though many of us were required to take health early on in school, it is overwhelming to look at designing your own exercise plan. That's why we'll be discussing the best practices for designing a workout plan for you, and even exploring a great alternative to traditional workout routines: yoga.

Managing diabetes is all about balance – however you look at it, you need to maintain a balance in your life in order to be able to fully control your diabetes. Whether it be balance in your blood-glucose levels, or balance in how you work out, it is the key word to your treatment.

A well-rounded exercise plan consists of many different types of workouts, each designed to focus on one particular trait or quality of your body.

Cardio

Cardiovascular activity is physical activity that is designed to get your heart pumping. As you breathe faster and deeper, your heart beats faster, and the oxygen in your bloodstream increases. The more often that you engage in cardiovascular activity, the more effectively your heart and lungs work.

This is especially important for those with diabetes, because high levels of blood-glucose can cause blood to circulate less efficiently, which is often what leads to some of the complications of diabetes. Regular cardiovascular activity directly combats this by circulating more oxygen-rich blood through the body more quickly.

According to the United States Department of Health, it is recommended that healthy adults get between 75 to 150 minutes of cardiovascular activity every week, depending on the intensity of the workout. This could be anything that gets your blood pumping quickly – for some, it may be running, and for others, it could be swimming. So long as your heart is pumping, you are doing it right.

Core Training

The muscles that are known as your core are located in your abdomen, lower back, and pelvis. Your core is the center of your body, where you coordinate movement between your upper and lower body. A stronger core means that your back becomes stronger and more protected from injury, while your own movements become more efficient.

Core exercise is any exercise that uses your core without support. One common core exercise, for example, is abdominal crunches.

Strength Training

Strength training is a type of training that actively works on strengthening your muscles and bones. It is used often in fields like body-building to increase muscle mass, but it is an important component of any well-rounded workout plan. It is suggested that you engage in strength training at least twice a week for full effectiveness.

Strength training exercises include pushups and squats, or even lifting weights.

Flexibility

Flexibility is a commonly overlooked component of well-balanced exercise routines, but it is no less important. Not only does being flexible contribute to your overall fitness level, it also prevents you from getting injured as often while working out or going about your day. Prior to any workout, it is important to stretch so that you do not hurt yourself.

Stretching also has many benefits for your health in the long-term, like ensuring that you will be able to more effectively for as long as possible in your life. It also helps your joints, posture, and even stress level. It is suggested that flexibility exercises are incorporated before or after the rest of the workout routine.

Balance

Similarly to flexibility, practicing balance is often an overlooked component of a good physical fitness program. However, the benefits of this particular type of training are clear – by practicing balance, you can stop yourself from being injured in much the same way that flexibility prevents injury during workouts. Balance is a much greater feature in physical activities such as dancing and yoga, but it is still something that should be incorporated into regular exercise programs. One exercise that's simple enough is just trying to stand on one leg for as long as possible.

Using Yoga to Exercise

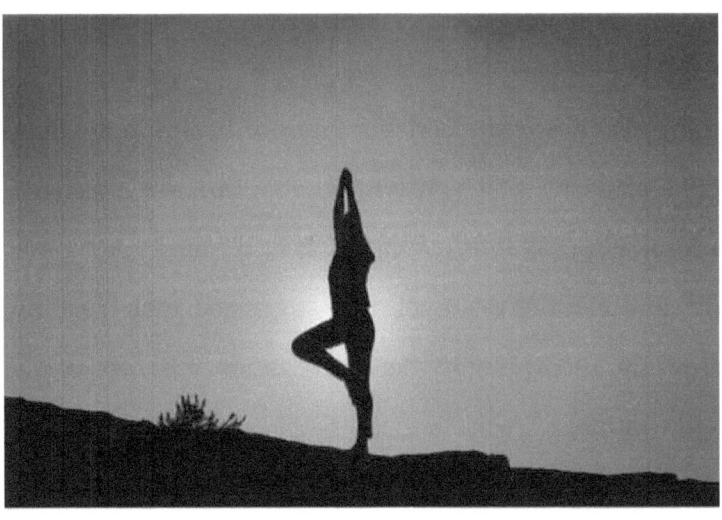

Yoga is a type of exercise that originated in India and is a common feature of Eastern religions such as Hinduism and Buddhism. However, because of its far-reaching health benefits, it is extremely popular today as a way to combat a number of health problems, whether they be mental or physical. Indeed, a large part of yoga is meditation, which we have already learned is also effective at maintaining a healthy lifestyle.

Because yoga is so relaxing, its physical benefits include lowering blood pressure, decreasing pain from arthritis or chronic pain, decreasing insomnia, and even getting rid of headaches. It is a great way for people who also juggle mental health problems to get in shape, because not only does it improve mood through the sheer fact that it is exercise, it also incorporates techniques from meditation, which cause it to be an extremely relaxing experience.

Yoga is primarily an exercise in flexibility and strength training, depending on the type and intensity of the yoga performed, but it can also fulfill other types of exercise. For example, hot yoga tends to be a much more intense experience of yoga, but it has its own set of benefits on top of regular yoga. You should choose a style of yoga that fits you more personally. If you are someone who has trouble with cardiovascular activity due to asthma, for example, regular yoga is a great option because it allows you to exercise without completely exhausting you or activating your asthma.

In fact, yoga has also been shown to increase circulation, despite the fact that it is not as heavy in cardiovascular exercise. This is because the relaxation techniques taught in yoga promote better circulation, which is again especially helpful for diabetics because of their already poor circulation.

There is also some evidence that yoga helps your body make better use of insulin because of the way that it decreases stress levels in your body. By decreasing cortisol and adrenaline, yoga can actually help increase how well insulin is used, enabling you to keep better track of your blood-glucose levels with diabetes.

You will also have better focus as it teaches you to focus on where your body is and how you are breathing. There are stories of very advanced practitioners of yoga even being able to have some control over their own nervous system by utilizing the meditation techniques found in yoga. In fact, combined with mindfulness, yoga is a great way to take control of your body and surroundings in order to combat diabetes.

There are many ways to get into practicing yoga, but the best experience by far is to start with a class or with videos. If you are not as interested in socializing, or feel embarrassed because you are a beginner with yoga, there are plenty of videos online to get into yoga. All you need is a mat and a large enough space to practice. If you are comfortable practicing yoga with others, research good yoga studios in your area, paying special attention to the instructors you'll be learning from. A good yoga instructor can be the key to really getting into the habit of yoga often.

Exercise, whether it be with yoga or a workout plan of your own design, is vitally important to the upkeep of diabetes. Even if you have not been diagnosed with the full-fledged disease, exercise in any form reduces your risk for diabetes, and can help you reverse its course if you are prediabetic. Making sure that you have a balanced and well-researched exercise plan is a great way to start to change your lifestyle.

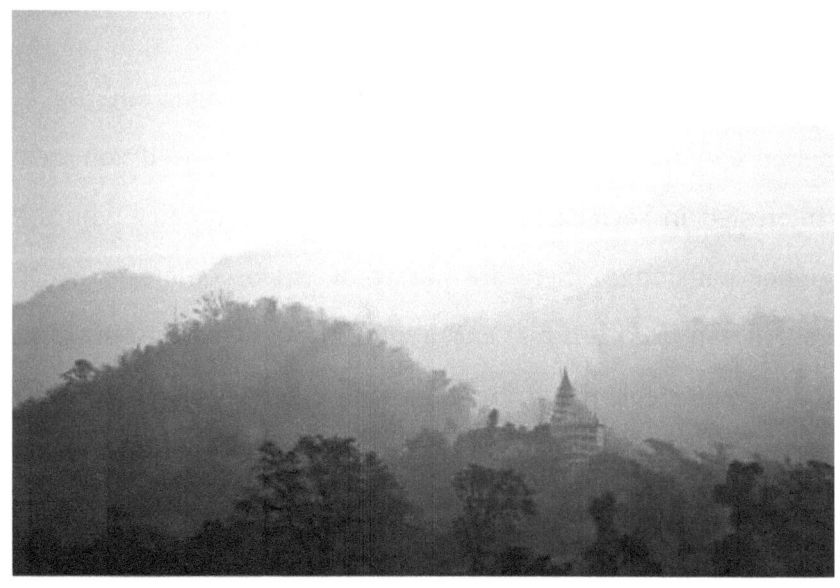

Chapter 5: Healthy Dieting for Diabetes

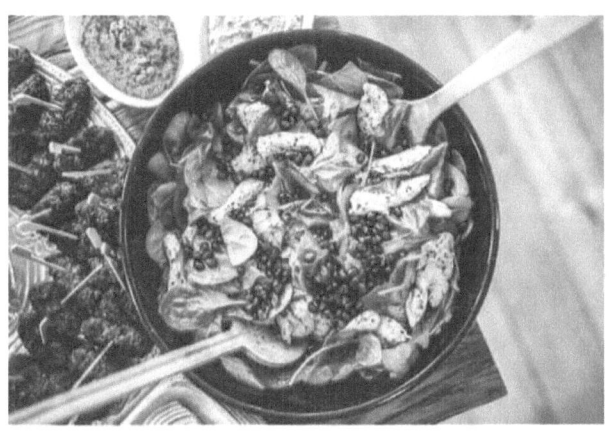

A healthy diet is often the best way to combat many different diseases and sicknesses, and diabetes is no different. Sticking, for example, to vegetables and fruit instead of overly sweet snacks has the added benefits of providing much-needed nutrients to your body. With a healthy diet, you feel better, happier, and lower your risk of diabetes.

Most dieting techniques for diabetes involves greatly decreasing portion sizes and sticking to food that is good for you instead of merely junk. Many people think that having diabetes means that they have to give up what they enjoy eating, which can feel like a punishment for having the disease. Happily, however, there is some evidence to suggest that there is another way where you can, metaphorically and literally, have your cake and eat it too.

Veganism is a diet in which people stop consuming animal products entirely. Unlike vegetarianism, it is much more strict because it does not allow for dairy products, or, really, anything that comes from an animal. It is a very popular diet in several different countries around the world, and even though it has become increasingly popular in the United States, it has yet to really take hold.

Its benefits for diabetes, though, are far-reaching. There is some evidence that shows that eating a diet derived mainly from plants (instead of meats and dairy), is a very effective way to combat the onset of diabetes. One study has even suggested that meat intake is actually correlated to insulin resistance. And since obesity is a large risk factor for diabetes, a vegan diet is a great way to lose weight and lower your risk for the disease as well, if you do not already have it.

Even if you do have it, however, you should consider veganism in order to combat it because it is a great way to keep track of what you are eating and slow down the onset. A vegan diet is very low in fatty foods, making it easy to lose weight. Many people are concerned with adopting this diet because they fear they will not get enough protein, but the fact of the matter is that humans do not necessarily need to have animal-derived protein in order to get enough protein. There is a great deal of protein in nuts and beans, which are prominent features in vegan diets.

In fact, animal-derived proteins may over time cause harm to the kidneys, especially for those who already have kidney damage. Plant-derived protein has far fewer health risks, and is often delicious.

In the rest of this chapter, you'll find an excellent collection of vegan recipes to help you get started maintaining your diet for diabetes. Each recipe lists both the serving size and the number of kilocalories in each recipe, and the recipes are sorted according to type. If you thought you had to give up your favorite sweets to manage your blood-glucose level, you were wrong. It is not totally necessary to give up your favorite foods if you are diabetic – by simply eating in moderation and sticking to a diet appropriate to your level of physical activity, age, and sex (whether you are on a 1200 kilocal per day diet or an 1800 kilocal per day diet), you can reverse the effects of diabetes as well.

Delicious Vegan Recipes for Diabetes

Breakfast

The first meal of the day is always the most important, breakfast is crucial and we have all been told this by everyone, from our mothers to our doctors; but somehow that still does not prevent some of us from either skipping breakfast entirely or opting for a less healthy breakfast. Here, you'll find a listing of totally vegan and delicious breakfast options that allow you to get the healthy calories you need without the danger of animal-derived products. Being diabetic certainly does not have to mean that you are required to skip some perfectly healthy pancakes, so long as you plan for them.

Vegan Pancakes (Kcal: 265)

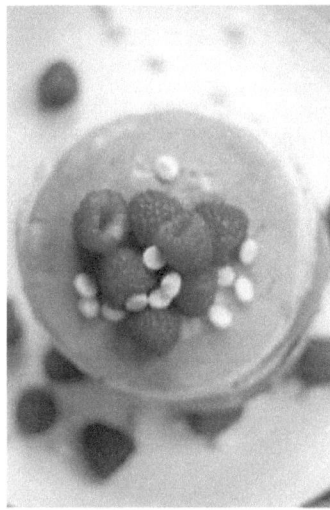

Servings: 3

Ingredients:

1 and 1/4 c. whole wheat flour

2 T. of beet sugar

2 t. of baking powder

1/2 teaspoon of salt

1 and 1/4 c. of water

1 T. of oil

Step 1:

In a large bowl, sift together the sugar, flour, baking soda, and salt.

Step 2:

In a different, small bowl, whisk together the water and the oil.

Step 3:

Slowly stir together the wet and dry ingredients until well-blended. The mixture will be lumpy. Do not overmix.

Step 4:

Over medium-high heat, heat the oil in a griddle. When it is heated and coats the bottom of the griddle, scoop batter and drop onto the griddle with large spoonfuls.

Step 5:

Cook pancakes until the edges are dry and the surface of the batter begins to bubble. Flip pancake, and cook other side until brown. Serve with preferred toppings.

***

Tofu Spinach Quiche (Kcal: 290)

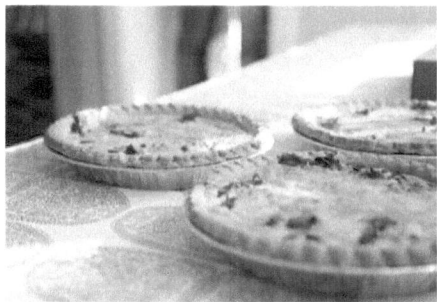

Servings: 6

Ingredients for Quiche:

1 vegan 9-inch pie crust, not baked

8 oz. of firm tofu

1/2 teaspoon of salt, plain

1/3 c. of almond milk, not sweetened

1 teaspoon of minced garlic

10 oz. of frozen thawed spinach, drained and chopped

1/2 teaspoon of pepper

1/2 c. of vegan Swiss-style cheese, shredded

1/4 c. of onion, diced

2/3 c. of cheddar-style cheese, vegan, shredded

Step 1:

You will need to allow your oven to heat up to 350°F beforehand.

Step 2:

Combine tofu and milk in a blender, mix until it is smooth. If necessary, more almond milk can be added. Blend in the salt and the pepper.

Step 3:

Mix these together in a bowl the spinach, garlic, onion, all the cheese, as well as your milk—tofu mixture and mix until well intermixed.

Step 4:

Dispense the mixture into the prepared pie crust. If you are unable to find a prepared vegan pie crust, there are many other recipes online.

Step 5:

Place quiche in the oven and then bake it for 30 minutes, or 'til the mixture is set, the top should look a light golden-brown color. Allow it to set for another five minutes or more before serving it.

***

Vegan Banana Muffins (Kcal: 450)

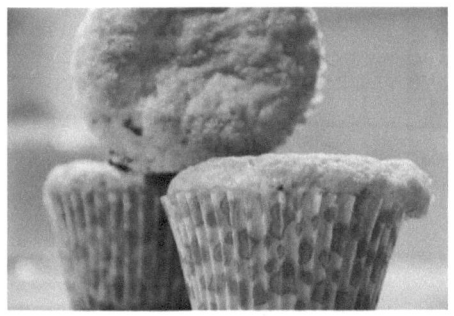

Servings: 12

Ingredients:

1 c. of coconut milk.

3 c. of whole wheat flour

1/2 c. of organic light brown sugar

1 teaspoon of salt

1 c. of beet sugar

2 c. of bananas, mashed

2 t. of baking powder

SAFE AND PROVEN DIABETES CURE

1 teaspoon of nutmeg, ground

1 c. of canola oil

1 teaspoon of baking soda

2 t. of cinnamon, ground

Step 1:

You will need to leave your oven on until it heats up until it reaches 350°F.

Step 2:

Use paper liners to line a 12-muffin pan or grease inside of muffin c.

Step 3:

Mix together the flour, brown sugar, baking soda, cinnamon, beet sugar, baking soda, salt and nutmeg in a sufficiently large container.

Step 4:

In a different container, stir the canola oil, coconut milk, and mashed bananas.

Step 5:

Slowly fold the banana mixture into the dry mix until it has all been properly assimilated and looks to be well combined.

Step 6:

Fill lined or greased muffin cups with banana and flour batter. Bake for 30 minutes. You can check that the muffins are ready by inserting a toothpick right in the middle of one of the muffins and checking if batter still sticks to it, if it comes out clean then you know the muffins are ready, if it does not, give it five more minutes.

***

Vegan Crepes (Kcal: 270)

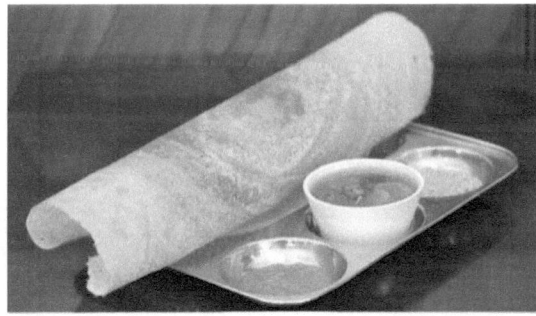

Servings: 4

SAFE AND PROVEN DIABETES CURE

Ingredients:

1/2 c. of water

1/4 c. of soy margarine, melted

1 T. of beet sugar

1/2 c. of soy milk

1 c. of whole wheat flour

1/4 teaspoon of salt

2 T. of maple syrup

Step 1:

Blend together soy milk, water, soy margarine, beet sugar, whole wheat flour, syrup, and salt in a sufficiently large container. You need the mixture to be thick so you must cover it and refrigerate it for a minimum of two hours.

Step 2:

Grease 6-inch skillet with the margarine, the bottom should be lightly covered with the grease so make sure you do not overdo it. You will know when the skillet is hot enough because all the margarine will melt.

Step 3:

Each crepe will need about three T. of batter. Before the margarine burns, pour the appropriate amount of batter into the skillet, swirl it until the bottom is completely coated with it. Cook crepe until golden brown before flipping and cooking on opposite side. Serve with your favorite toppings or fillings.

***

Cranberry-Orange Oatmeal (Kcal: 400)

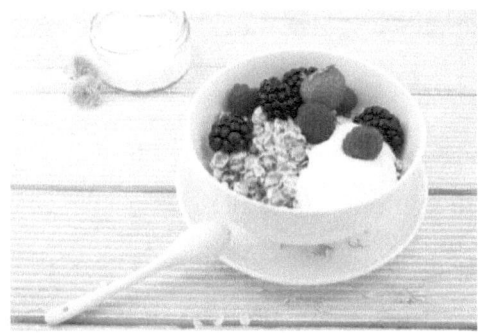

Servings: 1

Ingredients:

1/2 teaspoon of cinnamon, ground

1/4 teaspoon of turmeric, ground

3/4 c. of rolled oats

SAFE AND PROVEN DIABETES CURE

A pinch of ginger, ground

1/4 c. of cranberries, dried

1/2 c. of frozen blueberries

1 c. of water

1/4 c. of orange juice

Step 1:

In a microwave-safe dish, mix the old-fashioned rolled oats, cinnamon, cranberries, blueberries, turmeric, and ginger together. The cinnamon may be adjusted to taste preference. Stir to blend ingredients into a homogenous mixture.

Step 2:

Add water to mixture and stir together.

Step 3:

Microwave on high for two minutes, then stir in orange juice to preferred taste and consistency.

***

Avocado Toast (Kcal: 170)

Servings: 4

Ingredients:

4 slices of whole wheat bread

1 avocado, halved and pitted

1 ½ t. of olive oil, preferably extra-virgin

1/2 teaspoon of black pepper, ground

1/2 of a lemon, juiced

1/2 teaspoon of garlic powder

2 T. of fresh parsley, chopped

1/2 teaspoon of onion powder

1/2 teaspoon of salt

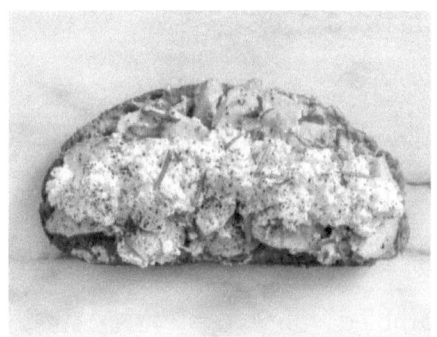

Step 1:

Toast bread according to your toaster or toaster oven's

instructions.

Step 2:

While the bread is toasting, scoop the avocado out of its skin and into a small bowl.

Step 3:

To the avocado add the order here specified the rest of the ingredients, meaning: olive oil, parsley, onion and garlic powder, lemon juice, salt, and pepper. Using a potato masher, blend together all ingredients. Spread over toast.

***

Eggless Tofu Scramble (Kcal: 200)

Servings: 2

Ingredients:

12 oz. of firm tofu, crumbled

1/2 c. of onion, diced

1/8 teaspoon of sea salt

1/4 c. of fresh shiitake mushrooms, diced

2 t. of vegetable oil

1/2 teaspoon of turmeric, ground

1/4 teaspoon of cumin, ground

1/4 c. of carrot, minced

Black pepper

Step 1:

Heat the vegetable oil over med. heat on a skillet. When hot, sauté the onions for two minutes or until it are soft.

Step 2:

To the onion in the pan, add carrot and continue to sauté for another two minutes or until the carrot is soft.

Step 3:

Add diced mushrooms to the pan as well and sauté for another two minutes.

Step 4:

Finally, add in tofu, cumin, and turmeric, then add salt and pepper to taste. Continue to sauté the mixture until the tofu is fully cooked, or another two minutes.

Soups & Sides

These small portions are great for snack or lunch, and the best part about them is that even though they're full of vegetables, they are still completely delicious and healthy. Here you'll find yummy soups for cold days or fun sides to serve at your next dinner party. People will hardly be able to believe that you are trying to manage diabetes.

Lentil Soup (Kcal: 350)

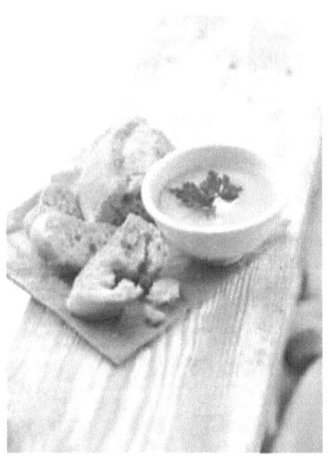

Servings: 6

Ingredients:

1 onion, chopped

1/4 c. of olive oil

2 carrots, diced

2 stalks of celery, chopped

2 cloves of garlic, minced

1 teaspoon of oregano, dried

1 bay leaf

1 teaspoon of basil, dried

1 14.5 oz. can of tomatoes, crushed

2 c. of lentils, dry

8 c. of vegetable broth

1/2 c. of spinach, rinsed and thinly sliced

2 T. of vinegar

Salt

Black pepper

Step 1:

Over medium heat, heat oil in a large soup pot.

Step 2:

Once oil is heated, add in carrots, onions, and celery. Cook the vegetables until soft.

Step 3:

Mix in bay leaf, basil, oregano, and garlic. Cooking should take around two minutes.

Step 4:

Stir in water, lentils, and tomatoes. Permit the entire mixture to begin to a boiling point before reducing the heat and allowing it to simmer for an hour.

Step 5:

Just before serving, add spinach to the soup pot and reduce the spinach.

Step 6:

Finally, stir in the salt, pepper, and vinegar to taste.

***

Black Bean Veggie Soup (Kcal: 165)

Servings: 8

Ingredients:

4 c. of vegetable broth, canned or homemade

2 15 oz. cans of black beans, rinsed and drained

1 T. of vegetable oil

1 med. size onion, chopped

1 garlic clove, minced

1 14.5 oz. can of tomatoes, stewed

2 carrots, chopped

1 teaspoon cumin, ground

2 t. of chili powder

1 8.75 oz. can of whole corn

1/4 teaspoon of black pepper, ground

Step 1:

In large saucepan and over medium heat, allow the vegetable oil to heat up. Make sure that the oil will cover the bottom of the saucepan.

Step 2:

Sauté garlic, carrots and onions together, toss constantly to prevent it from sticking and heat until the onion becomes soft., it should take five minutes.

Step 3:

Once the onion has softened and browned, add in the cumin and chili powder, continue to sauté for yet another minute.

Step 4:

Mix in the vegetable broth, corn, half of the beans, and pepper to the mixture, and boil.

Step 5:

While the vegetable mixture is boiling, puree the canned tomatoes and the second part of the beans. Once well-blended, add the entire vegetable and beans mixture to the cooking pot.

Step 6:

Permit it to simmer for ten to fifteen minutes by reducing the heat and covering the saucepan. Before turning off the heat, check that the carrots are soft.

***

Vegan Corn Chowder (Kcal: 150)

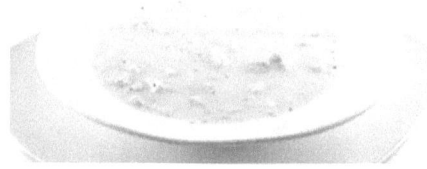

Servings: 6

Ingredients:

1 small onion, chopped

1 t. of garlic powder

2 T. of olive oil

1 T. of whole wheat flour

2 c. of corn

1 c. of carrots, chopped

2 c. of soy milk

1 c. of celery, chopped

1 clove of garlic, minced

SAFE AND PROVEN DIABETES CURE

1 teaspoon of parsley, dried

2 ½ of vegetable broth

1 teaspoon of salt

1 teaspoon of pepper

Step 1:

Allow the olive oil to heat up over medium heat and let it coat the bottom of a large skillet.

Step 2:

Sauté carrots, garlic, and onions, until the garlic becomes a golden-brown color.

Step 3:

In a separate pan, pour in vegetable broth and heat until warm. When the broth is warm enough, mix in the sautéed vegetables and the corn. If necessary, add water. You will know it is done when all the vegetables are soft.

Step 4:

Cut the heat down and stir in a c. of soy milk. Stir well before adding the second c. of soy milk.

Step 5:

Whisk flour into mixture, then stir in the salt, the pepper, and the garlic powder.

Step 6:

Cook for 15 to 20 minutes until the soup thickens.

***

Vegan Chili (Kcal: 390)

Servings: 8

Ingredients:

1 15 oz. can of red kidney beans, drained

1 15 oz. can of corn, whole kernel

1 T. of olive oil

2 bay leaves

1/2 medium onion, chopped

2 T. of oregano, dried

3 28 oz. cans of tomatoes, whole peeled, crushed

SAFE AND PROVEN DIABETES CURE

2 green bell peppers, chopped

1 teaspoon of cumin, ground

1 T. of salt

1/4 c. of chili powder

1 15 oz. can of black beans

2 celery stalks, finely chopped

2 12 oz. packages burger crumbles, vegan style

3 cloves of garlic, chopped

1 15 oz. can of garbanzo beans, drained

2 jalapeno peppers, chopped

2 4 oz. cans of green chili peppers, chopped, drained

1 T. of black pepper, ground

Step 1:

Warm the olive oil over medium heat in an appropriately large pot or saucepan, spread until the bottom of the pan is coated with it.

Step 2:

In the pot, add the onions, cumin, bay leaves, salt, and oregano. When the onion becomes tender and slightly brown you can add in garlic, jalapeño peppers, chili, green peppers, and celery.

Step 3:

Add the vegan butter crumbles when the vegetables are properly heated. Drop heat and then allow it to sit and simmer for five minutes, for this you will have to cover the pot.

Step 4:

After simmering the mixture, add the canned tomatoes. Add chili powder and pepper to taste.

Step 5:

Mix in black beans, kidney beans, and garbanzo beans. When it boils reduce the heat so it can simmer slowly. Set aside and permit it to sit for at least 45 minutes.

Step 6:

Add the corn while stirring. You should cook the whole thing together for around five extra minutes.

***

Hot-and-Sour Soup (Kcal: 240)

Servings: 4

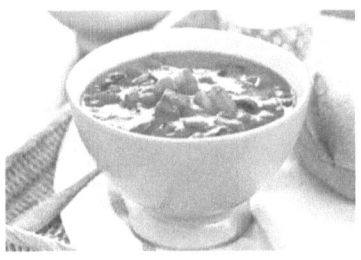

Ingredients:

4 shiitake mushrooms, dried

1 oz. of wood ear mushrooms, dried

2 c. of hot water

12 tiger lily buds, dried

3 T. of soy sauce

1/3 oz. of bamboo fungus

1/2 T. of chili oil

1/4 c. of cornstarch

5 T. of rice vinegar

8 oz. of firm tofu, cut into 1/4 inch strips

1 quart of vegetable broth

1/2 teaspoon of black pepper, ground

3/4 teaspoon of white pepper, ground

1/4 teaspoon of red pepper flakes, crushed

1/2 T. of sesame oil

1 c. of Chinese dried mushrooms

1 green onion, sliced

Step 1:

Soak shiitake mushrooms, wood mushrooms and lily buds in a bowl filled with hot but not boiling water. Let it sit for 20 minutes.

Step 2:

Once rehydrated, drain the bowl of water (reserving a small amount of the water), separate the stems and the mushroom head and slice them, then halve each of the lily buds.

Step 3:

In a different container, soak the fungus in ¼ of a c. of hot, salted water. Let it sit for 20 minutes, then drain and mince the fungus.

Step 4:

Blend the rice vinegar, soy sauce, and corn starch in a different container.

Add 1/2 tofu strips to the pot.

Step 5:

With the still warm water from rehydrating the mushrooms and lily buds, mix in the vegetable broth. Boil the water and broth.

Step 6:

Once the mixture has boiled, add in shiitake mushrooms, wood mushrooms, and lily buds. Lower the heat and then let it sit and simmer for 3-5 minutes.

Step 7:

While cooking, add white pepper, red pepper, and black pepper and stir together.

Step 8:

Mix the cornstarch with the remaining hot water in a different container. Slowly mix into the cooking broth mix until the entire soup has become thicker.

Step 9:

Finally, the tofu strips with the soy sauce in the saucepan and begin to boil again. Stir the bamboo fungus into the mixture, alongside the chili oil, sesame oil, and regular oil. You can use a green onion to garnish the dish.

***

Roasted Cauliflower Soup (Kcal: 140)

Servings: 6

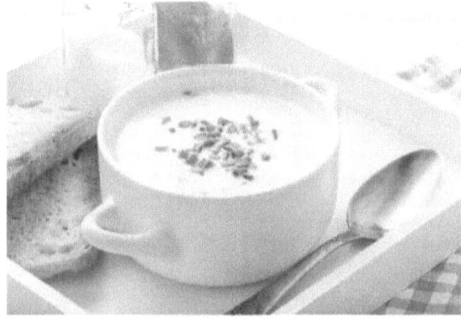

SAFE AND PROVEN DIABETES CURE

Ingredients:

Olive oil cooking spray

2 heads of cauliflower, pulled apart into florets

1/4 c. of olive oil

1 large onion, chopped

6 c. of water

Black pepper, ground

4 cloves of garlic, chopped

Salt

Step 1:

Soak the cauliflower florets in a container filled with slightly salted water. Set it aside and allow it to sit for 20 minutes.

Step 2:

After draining the bowl, arrange the cauliflower florets on your heavy aluminum foil sheet.

Step 3:

Lightly spray the cauliflower florets using the canned olive oil spray.

Step 4:

Preheat your broiler and place the rack six inches away from the heat-source.

Step 5:

Broil the cauliflower for 20 to 30 minutes. It should be browned before it is done.

Step 6:

Heat olive oil on a large pot until it coats the bottom of the pan. Sauté the onion until it becomes transparent, it should take around five minutes.

Step 7:

Stir in the brown cauliflower and garlic with the onions. Pour water into the pot and then season with black pepper and salt. Allow the mixture to simmer until the vegetables have become soft, it will take about 30 minutes

Step 8:

Blend the soup in the stockpot with an immersion hand blender. Take it up to a creamy consistency and serve.

***

Vegan Minestrone (Kcal: 320)

Servings: 4

Ingredients:

1 leek, sliced

3 T. of olive oil

2 carrots, which is chopped

1 zucchini, sliced thinly

4 oz. of green beans, cut into 1-inch size pieces

2 celery stalks, thinly sliced

1 and 1/2 quarts of vegetable broth

1 pound of tomatoes, chopped

1 T. of fresh thyme, chopped

1 15 oz. can cannellini beans, with the liquid

1/4 c. of elbow macaroni

Black pepper, ground

Salt

Step 1:

In a larger saucepan, warm up the olive oil over med heat until the oil completely coats the bottom of the pan.

Step 2:

Add in the leek, zucchini, carrots, green beans, and the celery to the olive oil in the pan, then cover and reduce the heat to low. Cook for 15 minutes, occasionally shaking the pan to stir-fry the vegetables.

Step 3:

Slowly add the vegetable broth, thyme, and tomatoes. Bring it to a boil at that point re-cover the pan. Reduce the heat to low and cook for 25-30 minutes.

Step 4:

Stir in cannellini beans (without draining the liquid) and the macaroni pasta. Cook for another 10 minutes, or until the pasta is at desired softness. Prior to serving, season with salt and pepper to taste.

Entrees

These delicious vegan entrees will have you questioning why you ever ate meat and dairy in the first place. Don't worry about being the odd one out at Thanksgiving dinner – with these dishes, you'll be able to fully enjoy your food and still be totally healthy. You'll even learn how to make a vegan "turkey" dinner.

Vegan Linguine with Mushrooms (Kcal: 430)

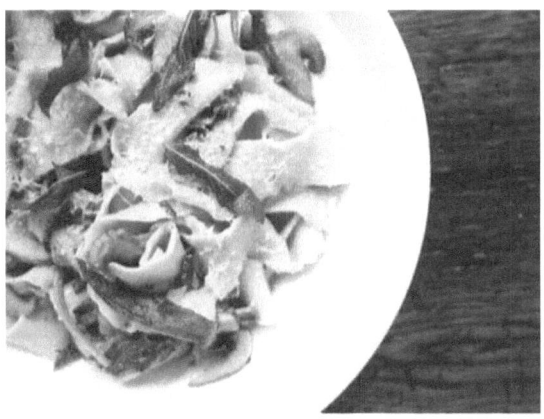

Servings: 6

Ingredients:

1 pound of uncooked linguine or fettuccine noodles

6 T. of olive oil

12 oz. of mushrooms, sliced thinly

3 cloves of garlic, chopped finely

¼ c. of nutritional yeast

2 green onions

¾ teaspoon of coarse-ground pepper

½ teaspoon of salt

Step 1:

Cook linguine according to directions on the box. Once linguine is fully cooked, drain all but ¾ of a c. of water. Place the pasta back into the pot.

Step 2:

While cooking the pasta, heat 6 T. of oil in a 12-inch skillet. Mix in the garlic and mushrooms. You will need to cook over medium, verging on high heat for around five minutes.

Step 3:

Toss the cooked noodles, mushrooms and garlic, nutritional yeast, salt, pepper, and ¾ c. of cooking water until well-mixed. Garnish or top with chopped green onion.

***

Vegan Thai Green Curry (Kcal: 540)

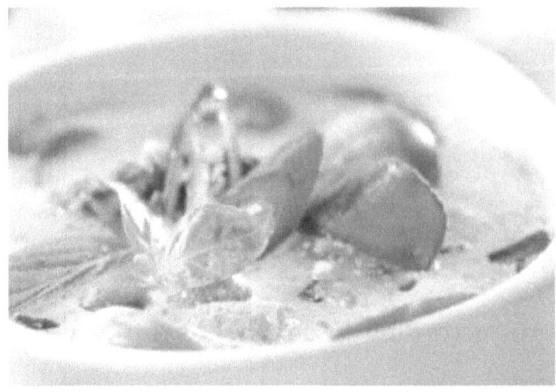

Servings: 4

Ingredients:

10 oz. of coconut milk

1 c. of uncooked basmati rice, rinsed

1 and ½ c. of water

14 oz. tofu, firm, pressed and cubed

3 T. of sesame oil

2 T. green curry paste

¼ teaspoon of salt

Step 1:

Stir together the rice and water in a medium saucepan. Once

boiling, lower the heat and let it sit and simmer while covered for 2o minutes, then remove from heat. Alternatively, cook rice using a rice cooker by following the its included instructions.

Step 2:

Heat 3 T. of sesame oil in a different saucepan and over medium heat. Mix in the cubed tofu. Pan fry tofu for 20 minutes until it is crisp and brown, stirring occasionally. Season with ¼ teaspoon of salt.

Step 3:

In yet another and smaller saucepan and over high heat allow the coconut milk to come up to a boil. Once boiling, mix in the green curry paste and mix until well-blended. Lower the heat until it is medium, verging on low, and simmer for 5 minutes. Top over cooked tofu and serve with rice.

***

Stuffed Tofurkey (Kcal: 470)

SAFE AND PROVEN DIABETES CURE

Servings: 10

Ingredients:

½ c. and 2 T. of sesame oil

1 and 1/3 c. of celery, diced

1 red onion, diced finely

80 oz. (5 packages) extra-firm tofu

2 cloves of garlic, minced

3 c. of stuffing (prepared in advance)

1 c. of mushrooms, chopped roughly

2 t. of dried thyme

1/8 c. of dried sage

¾ c. of tamari

1 and ½ t. of dried rosemary

2 T. of miso paste

½ teaspoon of orange zest

5 T. of orange juice

Fresh rosemary

1 teaspoon of honey mustard

Salt

Pepper

Step 1:

With a cheesecloth, line a round, medium-sized colander. Crumble tofu into colander, then mold into the shape of the colander. With another cheesecloth, cover the crumbled tofu, place a weight on top so that it presses down on it. TIP: Use a colander inside a large bowl so that it catches the liquid that presses out of the tofu.

Step 2:

Pour two T. of your preferred sesame oil into an appropriately-sized saucepan and allow it to heat up, spread it until it fully coats the bottom of the pan. Add sage, minced garlic, thyme, and ¼ c. of the tamari, rosemary, and pepper. Stir while cooking it for five minutes.

Step 3:

Before removing the pan from the heat mix the rest of the vegetables with the prepared stuffing.

Step 4:

You will need to allow your oven to heat up to 400°F as well as greasing a cookie sheet.

Step 5:

Combine ¼ c. tamari, ¼ c. of sesame oil, orange juice, miso, orange zest, and mustard in a small container. Mix the ingredients perfectly.

Step 6:

Remove the tofu from the fridge and take off the weight. Hollow it out until 1 in. of tofu is lining the mesh. Place what remains of the tofu in a separate container.

Step 7:

Brush over every little inch of the tofu lining using the miso seasoning and then scoop that into the middle of tofu shell. Place the excess tofu from the bowl, scoop out the leftovers, and arrange it at the top of the shell, over the stuffing.

Step 8:

Turn the colander upside-down carefully so that the stuffed tofurkey lies flat side down on the greased cookie sheet. Press the sides of the tofurkey to shape it more like a turkey, if you wish.

Step 9:

With ½ of your tamari and oil mixture brush the turkey, then add the rosemary on top of the tofu. You will have to bake for an hour after covering your turkey with foil.

Step 10:

After baking, take your turkey out of the oven and very carefully, so that you do not burn yourself, take off the aluminum. Now bathe the turkey in the rest of tamari mixture, just set aside four T. Now bake the turkey for another hour, when it is golden brown then you will know that it is done. Once transferred to an appropriate serving dish, brush the turkey with the remaining sauce.

***

Vegan Shepherd's Pie (Kcal: 550)

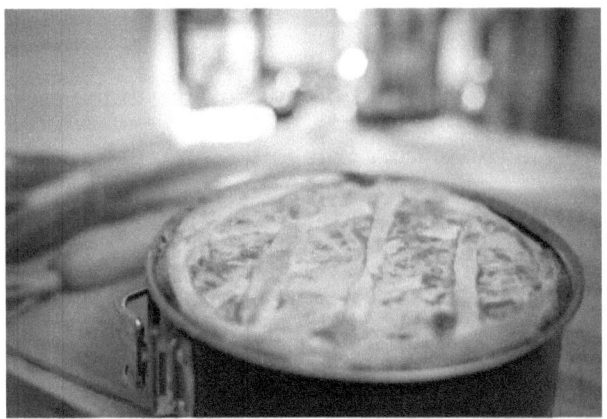

Servings: 6

Ingredients for top layer:

1/2 c. of vegan mayonnaise

5 russet Irish potatoes, peeled, cut into 1-inch cubes

1/2 c. of soymilk

3 T. of vegan cream cheese

1/4 c. of olive oil

2 t. of salt

Ingredients for the bottom layer:

1 large yellow onion, chopped

3 celery stalks, chopped

1 T. of vegetable oil

1 teaspoon of Italian seasoning

2 carrots, chopped

1 tomato, chopped

1 14-oz. package vegan ground beef

1/2 c. of peas, frozen

Black pepper

1 garlic clove, minced

1/2 c. vegan cheddar styled cheese, shredded

Step 1:

Add in the potatoes to a pot with water. Place over med heat, verging on high, heat until it starts boiling. Once it is boiling, lower the heat to medium-low and allow the potatoes to boil until they are softened. It should take around 25 minutes. Remove the water after the potatoes finish boiling.

Step 2:

Stir the soymilk, olive oil, vegan mayonnaise, salt, and vegan cream cheese together. This will act as a sauce so now this mixture into the potatoes.

Step 3:

With a potato masher, mash the whole thing until the entire mix is fluffy, smooth and without noticeable lumps. Set aside and heat up the oven to 400°F.

Step 4:

With cooking spray, spray a 2-quart baking dish.

Step 5:

Over medium heat and on a large skillet, warm the vegetable oil and allow it to cover the entire bottom of the pan. Cook the celery, carrots, onions, tomatoes, and peas for 10 minutes. You can check it is done by making sure that they have been softened. Stir occasionally.

Step 6:

Add the Italian seasoning, pepper, and garlic to the vegetables.

Step 7:

Lower the heat to medium, nearing, low. Pour the vegan style ground beef substitute into the vegetable's pan. For five minutes stir and break up the vegetarian ground beef, make sure that the whole mixture is hot.

Step 8:

Onto the greased baking dish spread the mixture. Add a layer of mashed potatoes over it, smooth them over with a tool. Add another layer by covering the top of the mashed potatoes with the cheese.

Step 9:

It should take around 20 minutes for the cheese to melt and brown slightly. Before removing make sure that the whole pie is hot.

***

Vegan Lasagna (Kcal: 510)

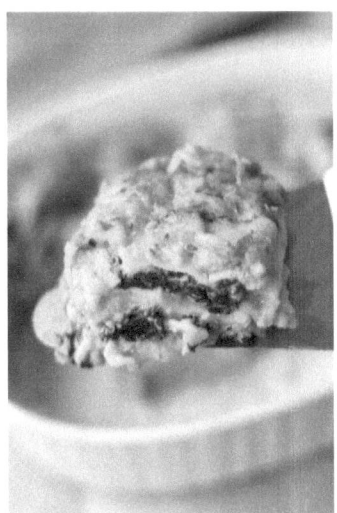

Servings: 8

Ingredients for the sauce:

3 T. of garlic, minced

1/3 c. of tomato paste

2 T. of olive oil

4 14.5 oz. cans stewed tomatoes

1 teaspoon of salt

1/2 of fresh parsley, chopped

1 t. of black pepper, ground

1/2 c. of fresh basil, chopped

Ingredients for the lasagna:

32 oz. of firm tofu

3 10 oz. packages of frozen spinach, thawed, drained and chopped

1/4 c. of fresh basil, chopped

1 16 oz. pkg. of lasagna noodles

2 T. of garlic, minced

1/2 teaspoon of salt

Black pepper to your taste

1/4 c. of fresh parsley, chopped

Directions for sauce:

Step 1:

Warm the olive oil in a large and thick saucepan over med-high heat, allow oil to coat the entire surface of the saucepan.

Step 2:

For 5 minutes, sauté the onions until they become tender and soft. Then mix in the garlic. You will need to cook this for five extra minutes.

Step 3:

Add the tomato paste, tomatoes, chopped parsley, and chopped basil to the saucepan. Make sure to mix the garlic and onion well before lowering the heat. Let it simmer by covering it and letting it sit for an hour, then add the salt and pepper, remember that you want to keep low sodium levels so do not overdo it.

Directions for the lasagna:

Step 1:

Boil a pot of salted water, it is advisable that you do it over high heat.. You will boil the lasagna noodles for at least 9 minutes but it is advisable that you check the package instructions just in case. When it's done pour the water out and rinse the lasagna noodles.

Step 2:

You will need to heat the oven first, 400°F will be enough.

Step 3:

Mash together the garlic, tofu, basil, salt, parsley and pepper in a large container. This is best done with your fingers or a potato mashing tool (or even a fork). Mix the ingredients well.

Step 4:

Use one c. of tomato sauce to cover the bare bottom of the casserole pan, and then place one layer of the boiled noodles on top. Add in a third of the tofu along the top of the noodle layer. Arrange the spinach evenly over the layer of tofu.

Step 5:

Now pour one and a half c. of the cooked sauce on top, then arrange another layer of lasagna and once again another portion of the tofu over this second layer, then top this tofu layer with another c. and a half of the tomato sauce. Finish off by covering the tomato sauce with your remaining lasagna noodles.

Step 6:

Cover the casserole with tinfoil and put inside the oven. Bake for 30-35 minutes.

***

Vegan Fajitas (Kcal: 200)

Servings: 6

Ingredients:

1/4 c. of olive oil

1/4 c. of red wine vinegar

1 teaspoon of oregano, dried

1 large onion, sliced

Salt

1 15 oz. can of black beans, drain it.

1 teaspoon of chili powder

Garlic salt

2 zucchinis, julienned

Pepper

1 teaspoon of beet sugar

2 yellow squash, julienned

1 red bell pepper, sliced

2 T. of olive oil

1 green bell pepper, sliced.

1 8.75 oz. can of corn, whole kernel, drain it

Step 1:

Mix the vinegar, olive oil, oregano, garlic salt, chili powder, beet sugar pepper, and salt in a large container.

Step 2:

Add the yellow squash, zucchini, green pepper, onion, and red pepper

to this marinade. Refrigerate for a minimum of half an hour to marinate the vegetables. Never go over 24 hours.

Step 3:

Allow the olive oil to heat up in a large skillet over medium heat. Make sure that the oil covers the entire bottom surface of the skillet.

Step 4:

When the vegetables are done marinating, drain them, and place them in the oil. Now, sauté until they become tender or for 10 to 15 minutes.

Step 5:

Stir in beans and corn. In order to brown the vegetables, you will need to sauté them over high heat. It should take five minutes. Serve.

***

Vegan Black Bean Burgers (Kcal: 265)

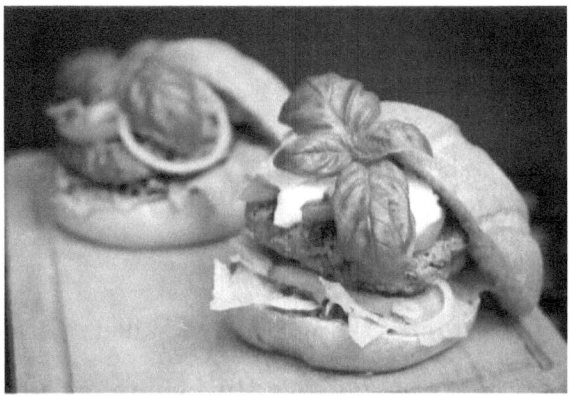

Servings: 4

Ingredients:

1 15 oz. can of black beans, drained and rinsed

1/3 c. of sweet onion, chopped

3 T. of chili-garlic sauce

3 baby carrots, grated

1 T. of cornstarch

1 T. of garlic, minced

2 slices of whole wheat bread, crumbled

1 T. of warm water

1 teaspoon of cumin, ground

1/4 c. green bell pepper, minced

1/4 teaspoon of salt

3/4 c. of whole wheat flour, as needed

1 teaspoon of chili powder

1/4 teaspoon of black pepper, ground

1 teaspoon of seafood seasoning

Step 1:

Grease a baking sheet and heat up the oven until it reaches 350°F.

Step 2:

Mash the black beans in a container, then add in the carrots, minced garlic, chopped onion, and minced bell pepper.

Step 3:

In a smaller bowl, mix together the chili-garlic sauce, water, cornstarch, seafood seasoning, cumin, pepper and salt. Fold this mix into the black beans.

Step 4:

Add the crumbled whole wheat bread to the black bean mixture and stir well. Add in whole wheat flour in increments of quarter c. into the black bean mixture until the batter is sticky.

Step 5:

Shape the black bean batter into patties that are about 3/4 of an inch thick.

Step 6:

The patties will have to be baked for 10 minutes on each side. It is better that the patty is brown and thoroughly cooked. Serve with vegan buns and your preferred toppings.

***

Tofu Skewers (Kcal: 300)

Servings: 2

Ingredients:

1 zucchini, cut into skewer-size chunks

8 oz. of extra-firm tofu, pressed sliced into skewer-size chunks

10 large mushrooms

1 red bell pepper, sliced into skewer-size chunks

2 T. of sesame oil

1/4 c. of soy sauce

2 T. of chili-garlic sauce

Black pepper

1/4 c. of onion, diced

1 jalapeno pepper, diced

Step 1:

Mix together the chili–garlic sauce, the soy sauce, the sesame oil, onions, pepper, and jalapeño in a small container.

Step 2:

Place the chunks of tofu and vegetables in a separate small container. Pour the sauce mixt on top of the chunks, then toss lightly so that all chunks are lightly coated with the sauce.

Step 3:

Cover the chunked vegetables and tofu. Marinate for at least one hour in the refrigerator.

Step 4:

Take the grate of an outdoor grill and preheat to medium-high heat after oiling it lightly.

Step 5:

Skewer the marinated and chunked tofu and vegetables. Grill the skewers for 10 minutes each, or to preferred level of doneness. The remaining marinade can be used as a dipping sauce.

***

Mac and Cheese (Kcal: 650)

Servings: 4

Ingredients:

1 c. of cashews

1/3 c. of canola oil

Salt

1 medium onion, chopped

1 8 oz. package of elbow macaroni

1 and 1/3 c. of water

1/3 c. of lemon juice

1 T. of vegetable oil

1 teaspoon of garlic powder

3 T. of nutritional yeast

4 oz. of roasted red peppers, drained

1 teaspoon of onion powder

Step 1:

You will need to allow your oven to heat up to 350°F beforehand.

Step 2:

Boil a large pot of lightly salted water, then add uncooked macaroni elbows. Cook 8 to 10 minutes (or according to package directions) until the noodles are at the desired level of softness. Drain the noodles, then transfer them to a medium baking dish.

Step 3:

In a medium-sized saucepan over medium heat, heat the vegetable oil until it coats the bottom of the pan. Stir in the onion and sauté until lightly browned. Gently mix the cooked onion with the cooked macaroni noodles.

Step 4:

Mix cashews, lemon juice, water, and salt in a blender or a food processor until well-mixed. Gradually add to this mixture the canola oil, roasted red peppers, nutritional yeast, garlic powder, and onion powder until all ingredients are smooth.

Step 5:

Thoroughly mix the blended ingredients with the mixed macaroni and onions, then bake for 45 minutes in the oven, until lightly browned. Allow the dish to cool for 10 to 15 minutes before serving.

Desserts

Being diabetic does not necessarily have to mean that you give up all desserts. In fact, you can easily enjoy some dessert so long as it is eaten in moderation and you monitor your blood-glucose level carefully. Here is just a small sampling of how you can create delicious vegan desserts. Because all of these recipes are vegan, they are a much better option for dessert so you do not have to give up on the tasty foods you love because of diabetes.

Vegan Brownies (Kcal: 285)

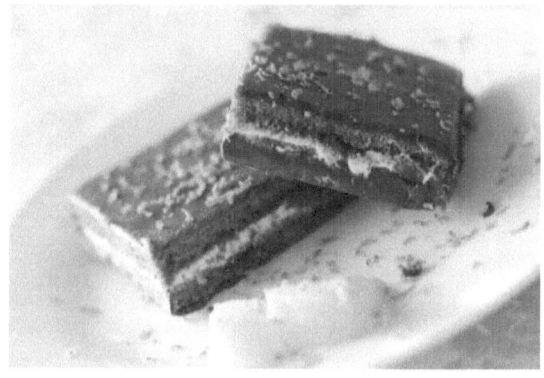

Servings: 16

Ingredients:

2 c. of whole wheat flour

3/4 c. of unsweetened cocoa powder

2 c. of beet sugar

SAFE AND PROVEN DIABETES CURE

1 teaspoon of baking powder

1 teaspoon of salt

1 teaspoon of vanilla extract

1 c. of water

1 c. of vegetable oil

Step 1:

You will need to allow your oven to heat up to 350°F beforehand.

Step 2:

In a mixing container, stir the whole wheat flour, baking powder, beet sugar, salt and unsweetened cocoa powder.

Step 3:

Add vegetable oil, vanilla extract, and water to the dry ingredients. Blend them together by mixing thoroughly. To ensure that everything is cooked evenly you will have to make sure that the batter is spread evenly.

Step 4:

Bake the brownies for 30 minutes. You will know that they

are done when the top of the mixture is no longer shiny. Allow to cool on the counter for a minimum of ten minutes before you eat or cut them.

***

Tofu Pumpkin Pie (Kcal: 230)

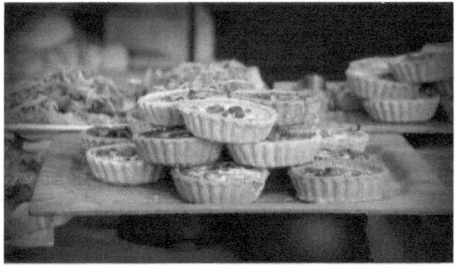

Servings: 8

Ingredients:

1 9-inch unbaked vegan pie crust

10.5 oz. of silken tofu, pressed

1 16 oz. can of pumpkin puree

1/2 teaspoon of ginger, ground

1 teaspoon of cinnamon, ground

1/4 teaspoon of cloves, ground

1/2 teaspoon of salt

3/4 c. of beet sugar

Step 1:

Puree the tofu, pumpkin, sugar, salt, cinnamon, ginger, and clove using a blender on a slow speed, the mixture should be smooth and without lumps. Add the mixture on top of the pie crust. Allow the oven to heat up until it reaches 450°F.

Step 2:

Bake the pie for 15 minutes. The you will need to reduce the heat of the oven by turning it down to 350°F, bake for 40 more minutes and check that it is done by pressing a toothpick into the center of the pie, if it comes without any batter, then it means that it is done. Cool on the counter before serving.

***

Avocado Pudding (Kcal: 400)

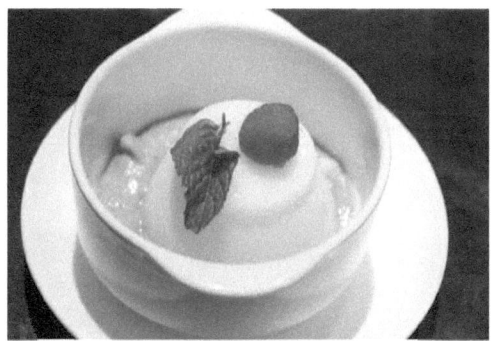

Servings: 4

Ingredients:

1/2 c. of organic light brown sugar

1/3 c. of coconut milk

2 large avocados, pitted and cubed

1/2 c. of unsweetened cocoa powder

1 pinch of cinnamon, ground

2 t. of vanilla extract

Step 1:

Use either a food processor or a blende to blend all the ingredients until they become smooth and lump-free.

Step 2:

Chill blended mixture for about 30 minutes before serving.

***

Roasted Almond Cookies (Kcal: 270)

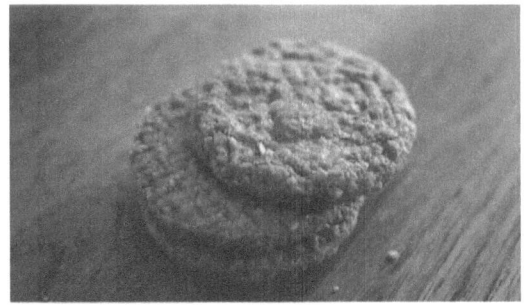

Servings: 6

Ingredients:

1 teaspoon of almond extract

1 c. of whole almonds, raw

1 c. of oat flour

1/2 c. of maple syrup

Step 1:

Allow your oven to heat up to 275 ° F.

Step 2:

After spreading the whole and raw almonds onto a baking sheet, toast them until the nuts become fragrant and begin to turn a nice golden brown color. This should take about 45 minutes. They burn very quickly if they are not watched.

Step 3:

Once the almonds are toasted, set them aside to cool down until their they are at room temperature. To finely blend the roasted almonds you can use either a blender or a food processor.

Step 4:

You will have to grease a baking sheet with baking oil or vegetable oil.

Step 5:

Increase the oven's temperature until it reaches 350°F.

Step 6:

In a sizeable mixing bowl, mix simultaneously the blended almonds, maple syrup, oat flour, and almond extract.

Step 7:

Separate the mixture into six even-sized balls, then flatten them onto the baking sheet as cookies that are about 1/4 inch thick.

Step 8:

Place the cookies inside the oven and bake them for 15 minutes, you can check to see if they are done by checking if they are crisp and brown around the edges. Much like the roasted almonds, they will burn quite easily if they are not watched. Once baked, take them out of the oven and let them cool before you eat them

***

Even though it is tough for anyone to follow such a strict diet and exercise program, eating vegan and trying to fit in physical activity is an excellent way to combat the onset of diabetes. Much like the women that Dr. Christopher J. Davies treated, you too can begin to reverse the effects of diabetes on your body with healthy lifestyle habits. So long as you stay motivated and set goals for yourself, you will still be able to live out a full and happy life, even with diabetes.

Conclusion

Thank for making it through to the end of *Safe and Proven Diabetes Cure*. We hope that it was an effective tool in demystifying diabetes and providing you with the knowledge you need to maintain your disease.

The next step is to keep practicing what you have learned and live out your life fully, even with diabetes. Even though it is a serious diagnosis, it does not have to be the end of the world. By staying knowledgeable and maintaining a better lifestyle, you can reverse your diabetes too. Whether you decide to create your own unique workout plan following the guidelines for balance in this book, or do yoga, or meditate, or even eat vegan, you can help yourself get better.

Finally, if you found this book useful in anyway, a review on Amazon is always appreciated!